That's Not My Cat

Anne-Marie Tucker

with Candace J. Semien

Illustrations by Nai Saechao

That's Not My Cat

Anne-Marie Tucker

with Candace J. Semien

The Tony Meduri TBI Fund, Inc., a 501c3 non-profit organization
904-200-1130 ~ http://www.tbifundinc.com

Editing by Candace J. Semien
Book Design by Jozef Syndicate www.JozefSyndicate.com
Illustrations by Nai Saechao

ISBN 978-1-944155-31-5
Library of Congress Control Number: 2022943884

Sometimes the people we love, our family or friends, change because of circumstances beyond their control. This could happen if they were involved in a tragic accident, suffered life-altering injuries, or due to a medical reason such as a stroke, disease, or illness.

Pop Pop was one of those people. He was in a car accident that resulted in a traumatic brain injury and caused life-altering injuries. He was no longer the father, grandfather, son, or person we once knew. As the years passed, his brain injury evolved into dementia, which meant he would sometimes forget things, events, and even people like me—his daughter.

After years of caring for my father, I found inspiration for this book. Due to Pop Pop's dementia, I thought a pet would be a good distraction for him and fun for us. Each day, we visited him and Blaze, the cat. No matter what, Blaze gave us something to smile about and every day Pop Pop would tell us, "That's not my cat!". We all found humor in the situation.

This book is written for all the grandsons, granddaughters, children, brothers, sisters, parents, and caregivers who have loved someone with all their heart, regardless injury, illness, or disability.

When you have a situation like mine, it is important to embrace the new person and make new memories with them. Life is full of obstacles and many of which are unexpected. We can never imagine our own mom or dad being different or forgetting who we are.

So dive in, stay positive, stay strong, talk about how you are feeling, and most importantly, keep loving them.

— Anne-Marie

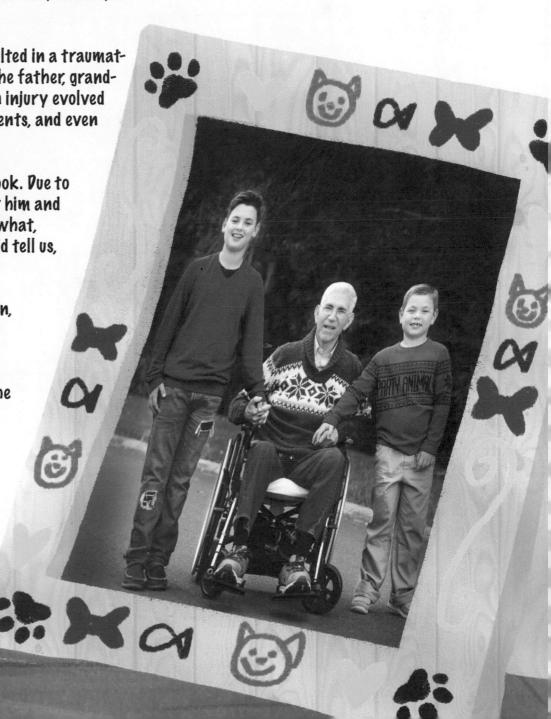

"What a cute kitty!
Who does he belong to?"
Pop Pop asks curiously.

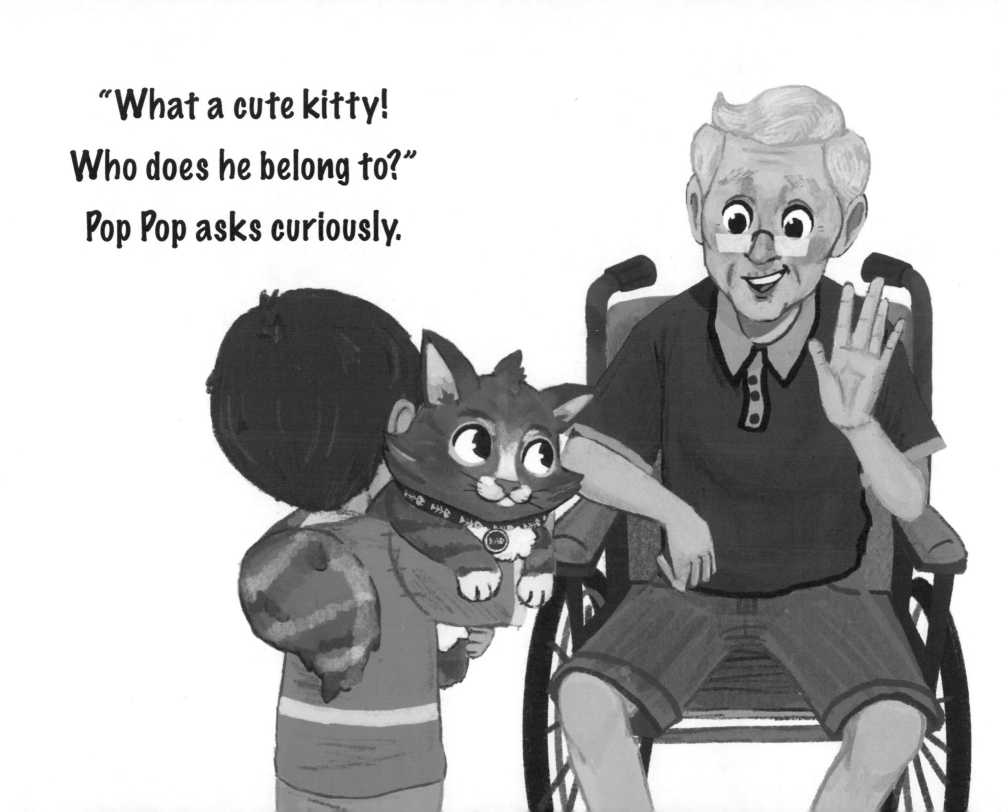

"You are funny, Pop Pop."

Chase smiles and says to his grandfather.

"Blaze is your kitty!

He has been living with you for a long time."

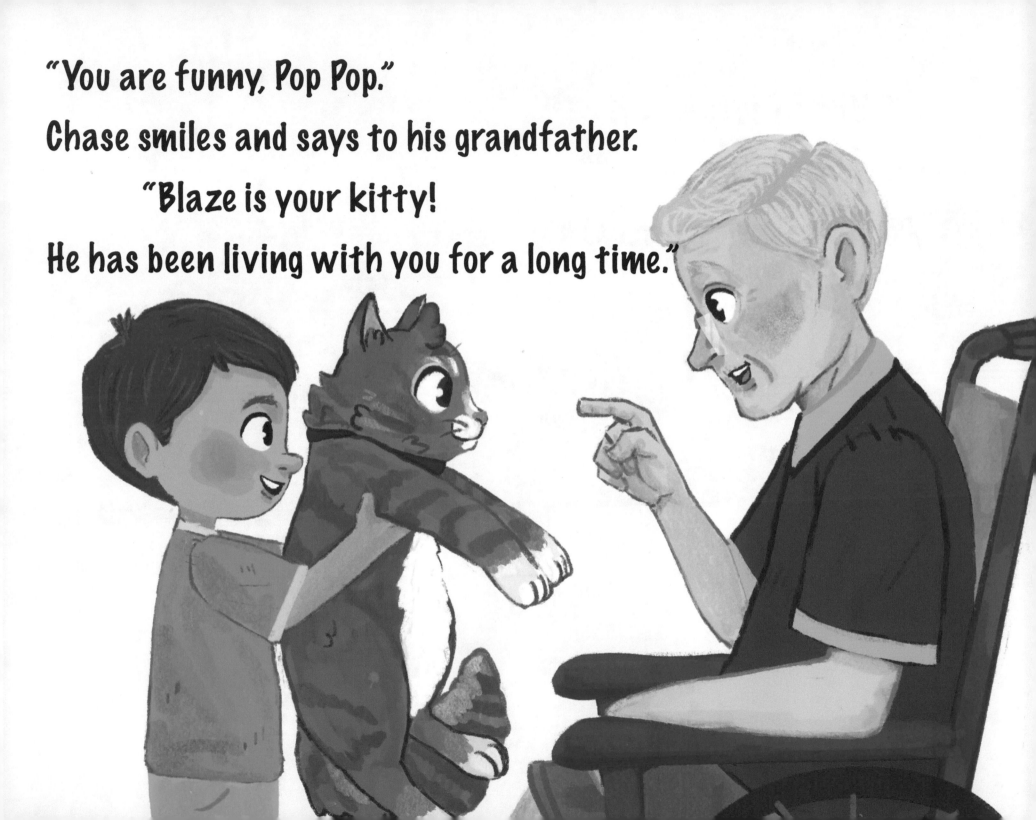

"Nope! That's Not My Cat!
I don't like cats!"
Pop Pop proclaims.

"Well, Pop Pop, Blaze is your cat.

He lives here and you like him.

He keeps you and the caregivers company.

And most of all, I like to play with him

when I come to visit you," says Chase.

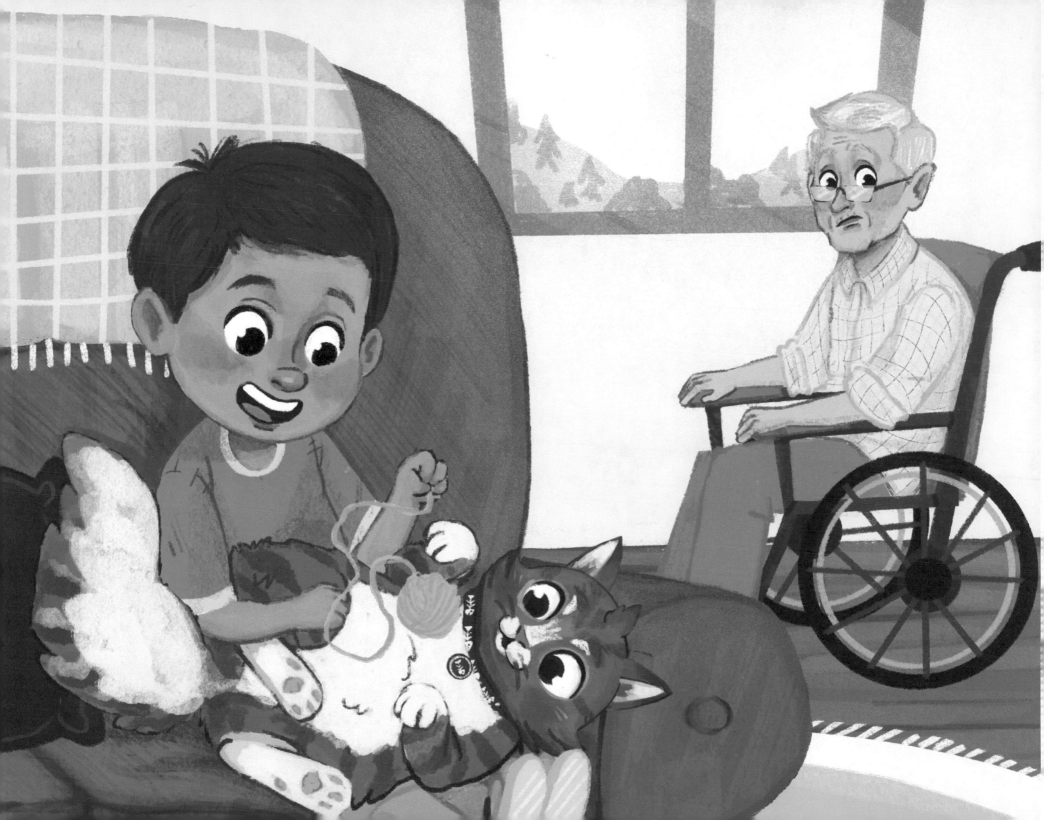

"We adopted Blaze from the animal shelter. Don't you remember?" Chase looks at Pop Pop in wonder.

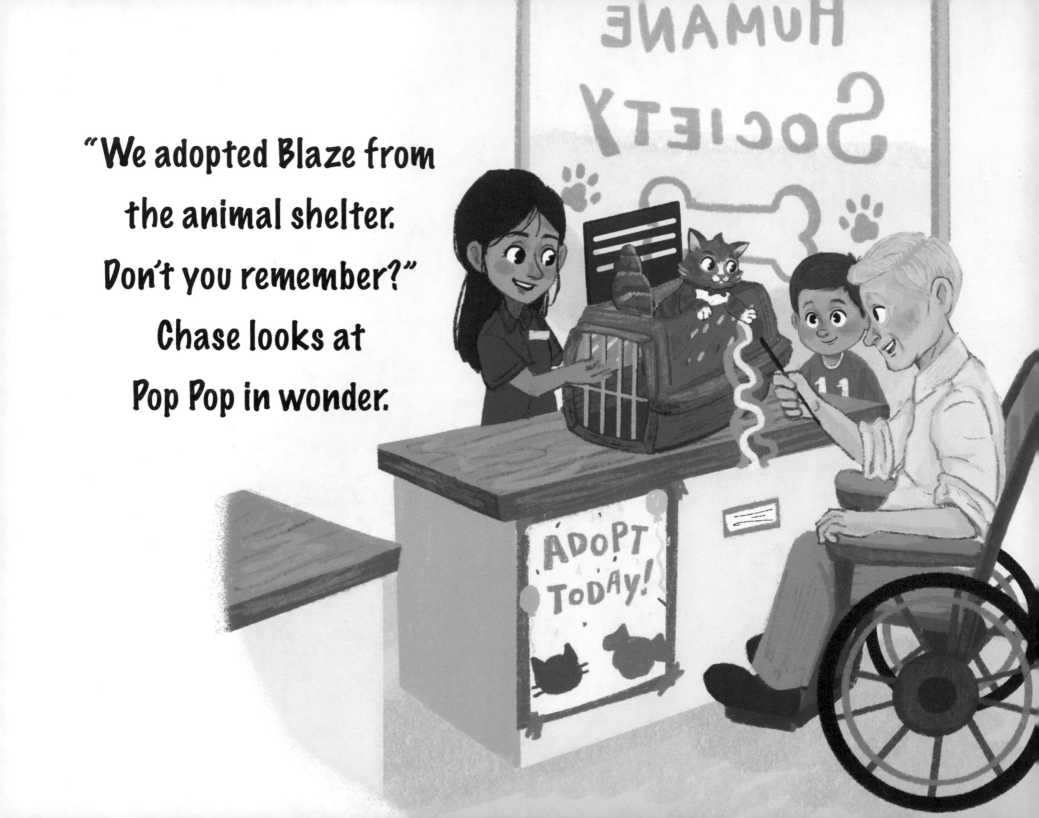

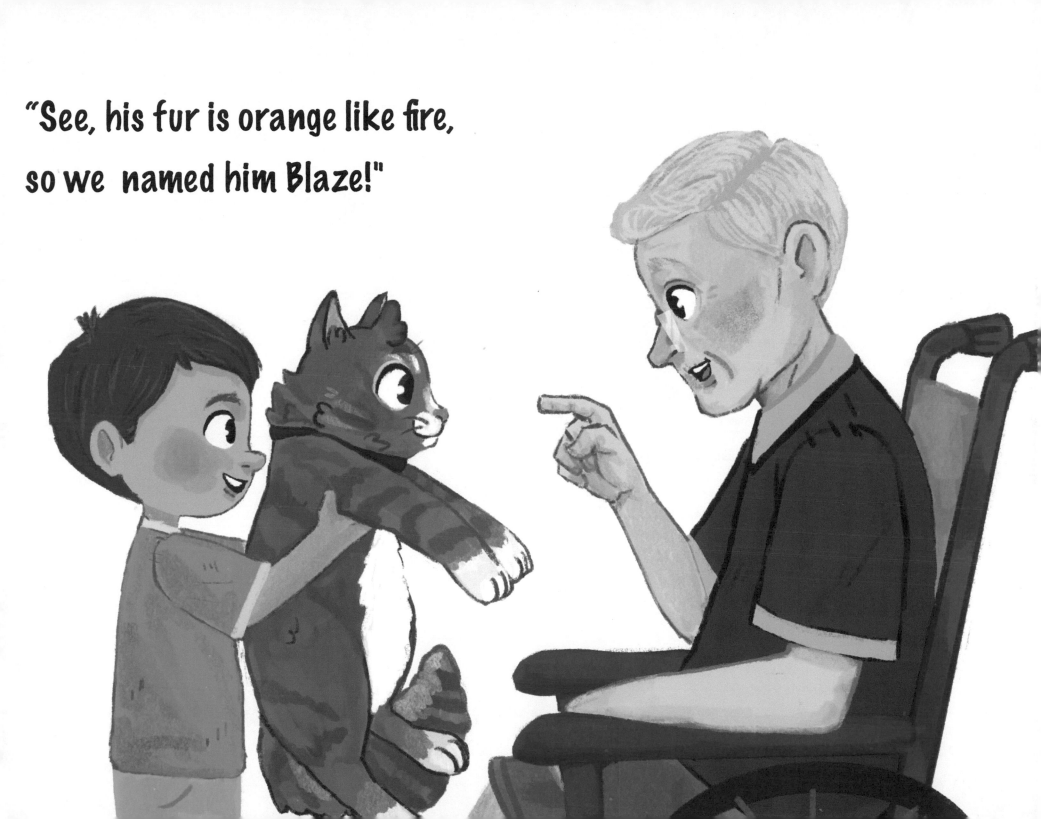

"See, his fur is orange like fire, so we named him Blaze!"

Pop Pop shakes his head.
"Nope, That's not my cat!"

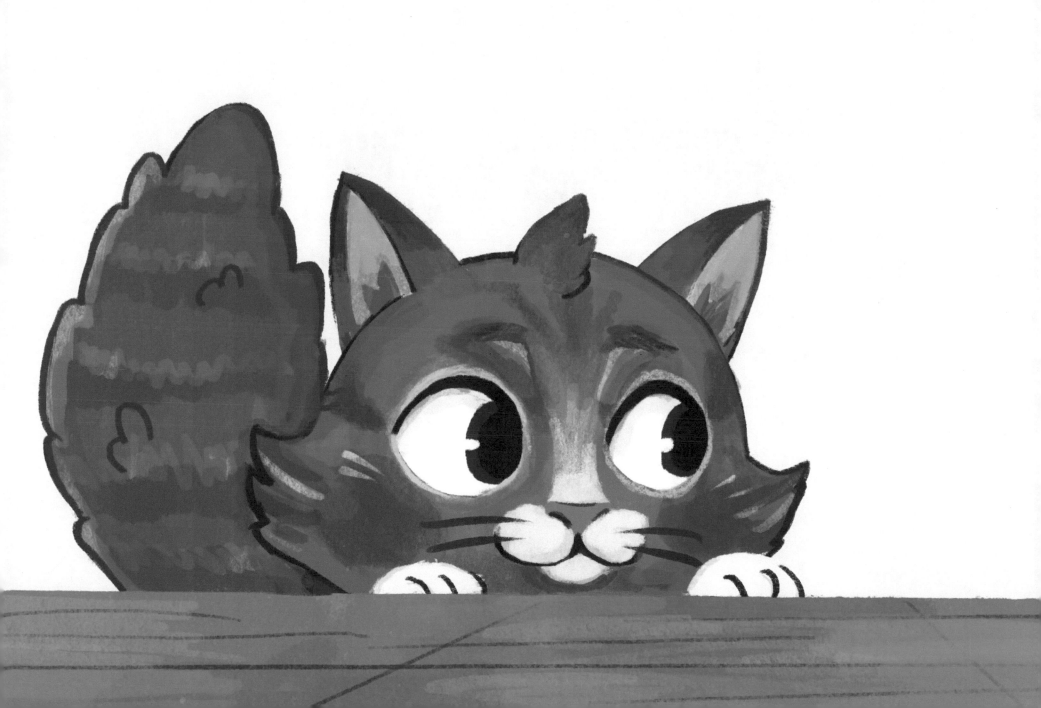

When Mom walks into the room,
Chase asks,
"Mom, why doesn't Pop Pop
remember things sometimes?"
Mom replies gently,
"Well, Pop Pop had a brain injury from a car accident,
and now he has dementia."

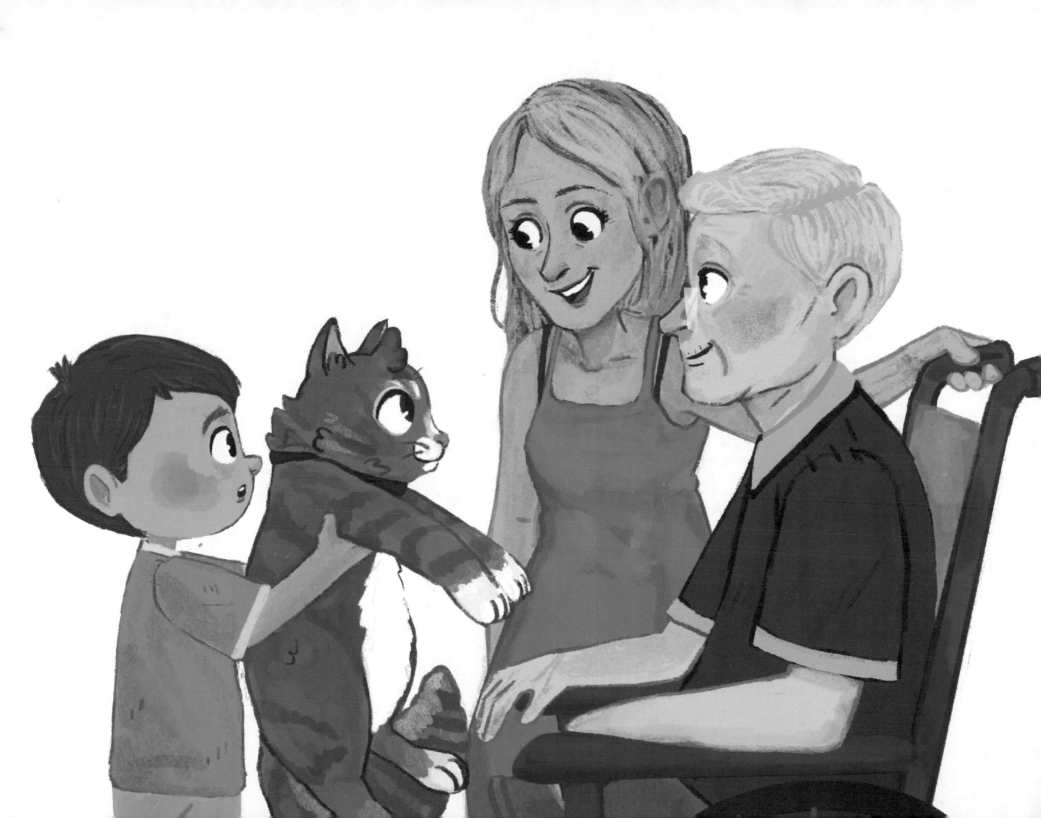

"Dementia is an illness that can cause people
to forget things sometimes.
They can even forget things and people closest to them,
like family and pets.
Just like Pop Pop forgets us sometimes
and he forgets that Blaze is his pet."

Chase looks very concerned
and Mom continues to explain.

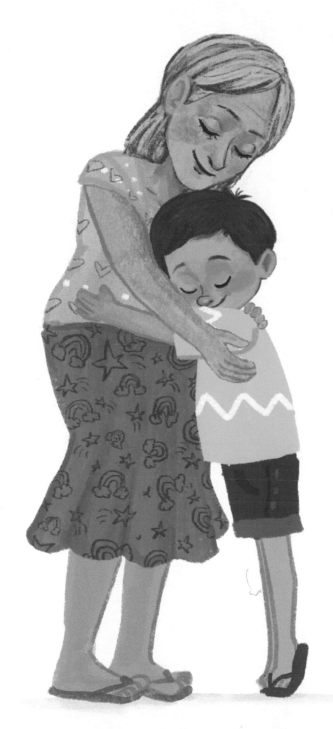

"Even though Pop Pop's dementia and brain injury may cause him to forget things, alot of times, he still remembers. And guess what else!

Blaze knows in his heart that Pop Pop loves him!"

Mom gives Chase a big hug and says, "And we know that Pop Pop loves us, too. Even when he can't remember who we are sometimes."

Chase scratches his chin and thinks
"I have to help Pop Pop remember, but how?"

Then, he says,
"Pop Pop, don't you remember
how Blaze loves to watch you eat and he sits with you
at the table?"

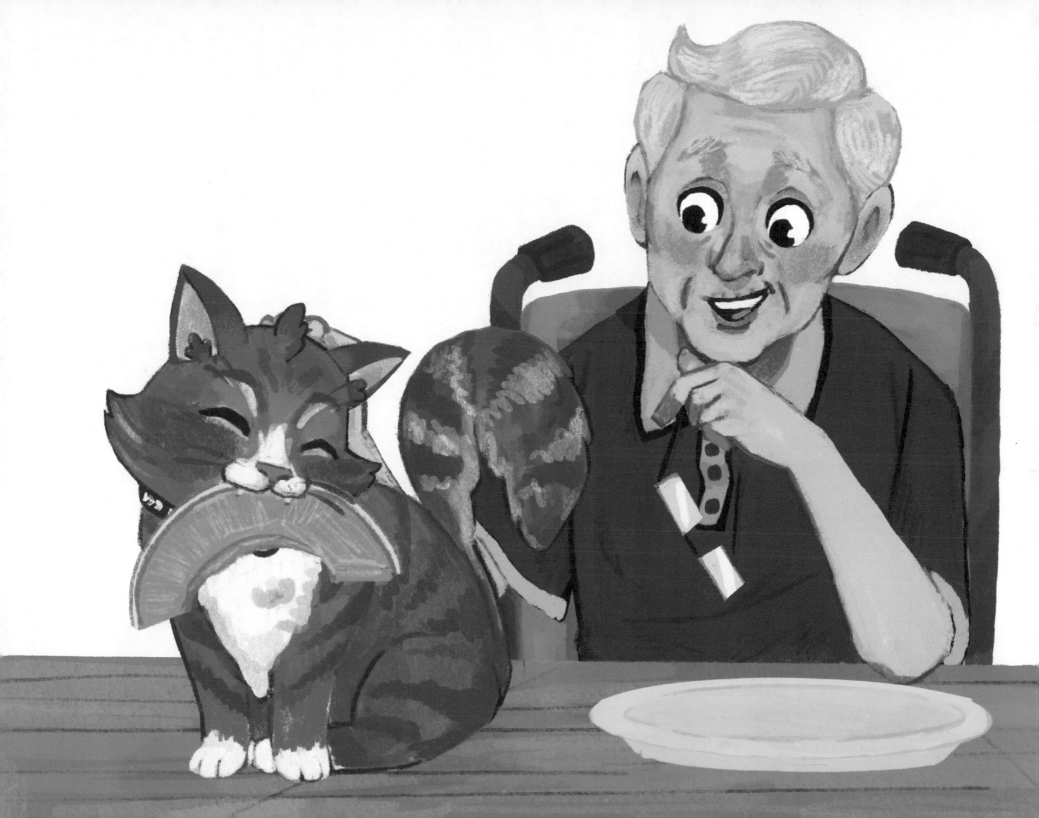

"Nope," Pop Pop says,
"Nope, That's not my cat!"

"But, Pop Pop! "
Chase tries again to get Pop Pop to remember.

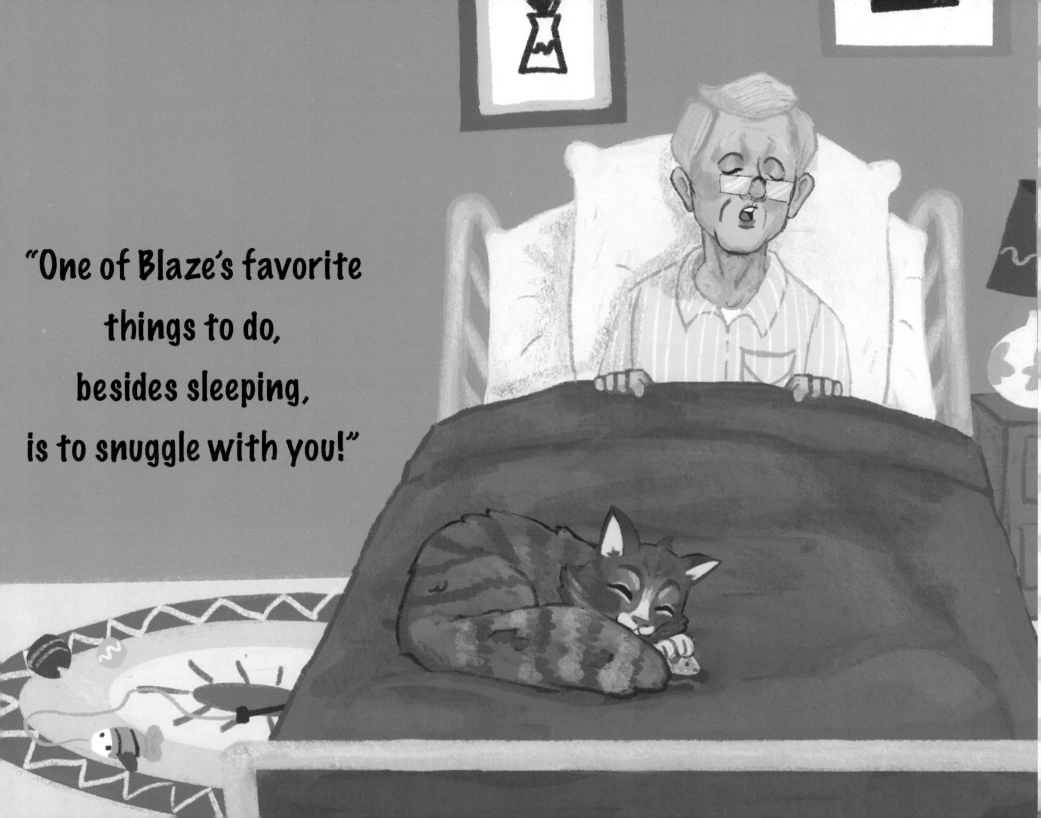

"One of Blaze's favorite things to do, besides sleeping, is to snuggle with you!"

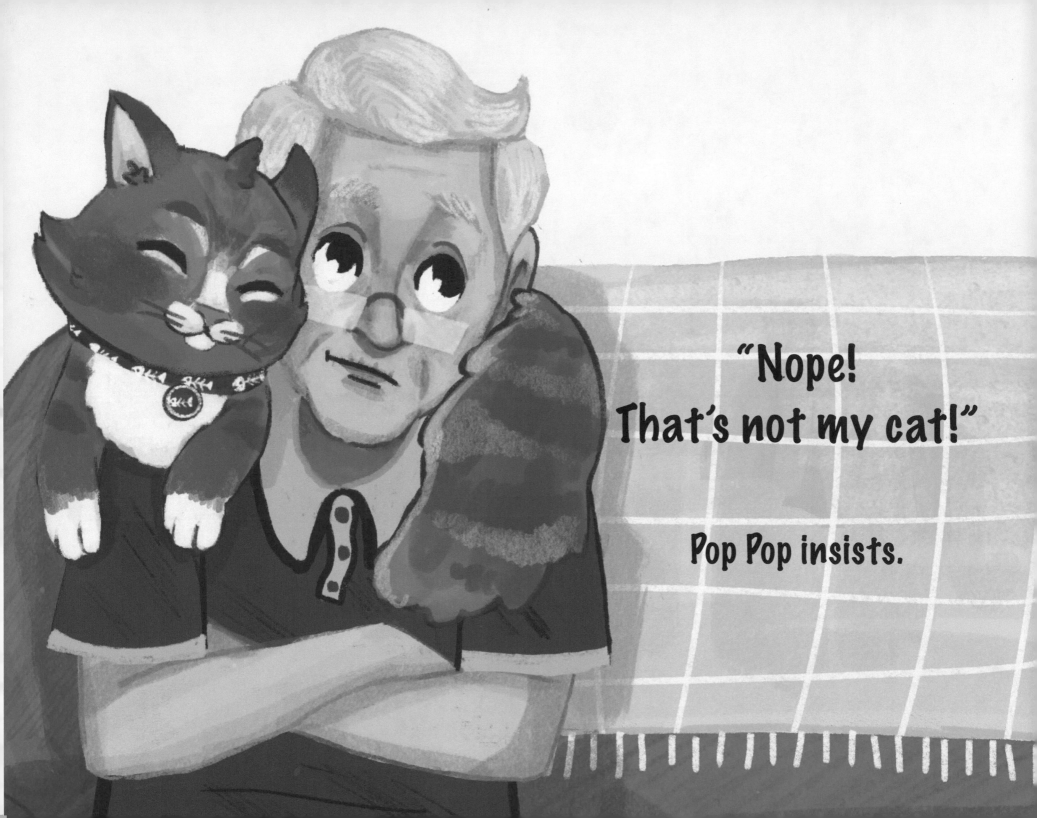

"Nope!
That's not my cat!"

Pop Pop insists.

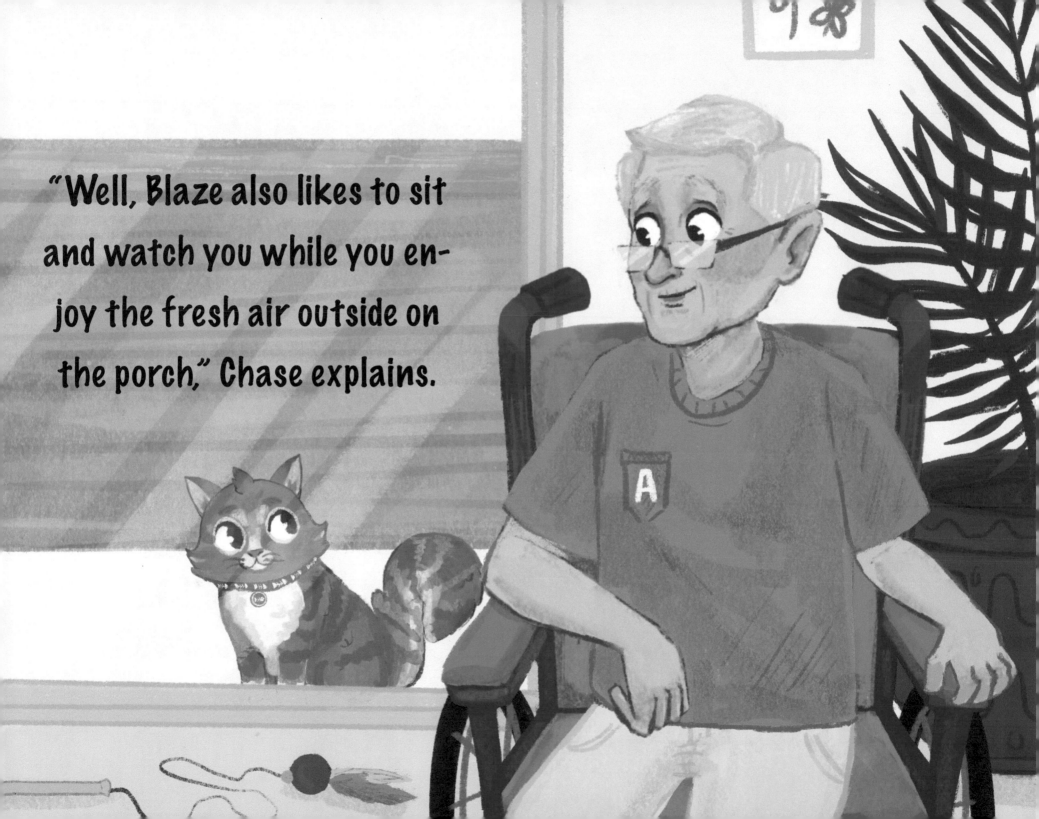

"Well, Blaze also likes to sit and watch you while you enjoy the fresh air outside on the porch," Chase explains.

"Nope! That's not my cat!"

Pop Pop is getting angry, but Chase continues.

"What about when Blaze likes to eat your favorite snack,
CANTALOUPE!

He always steals it off your plate!"

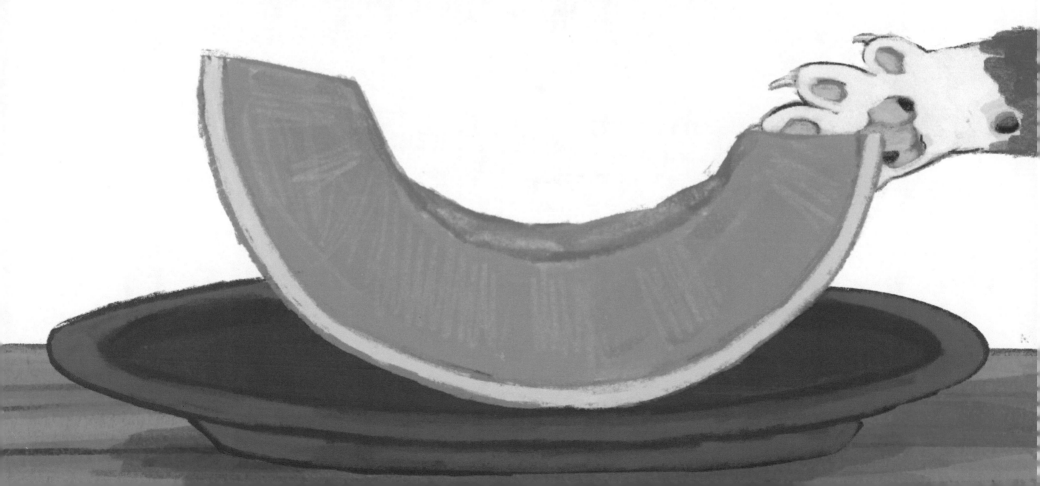

"Don't you remember that?"

Chase asks.

He smiles and thinks,

"Pop Pop will surely remember that! "

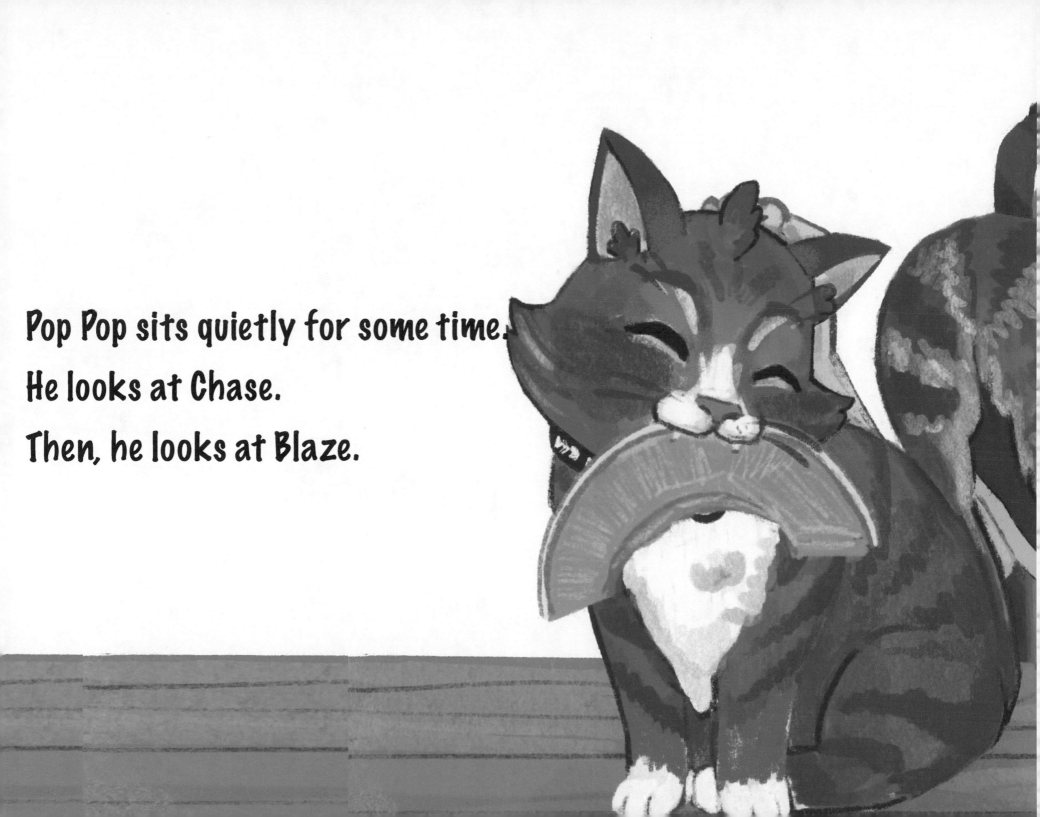

Pop Pop sits quietly for some time.

He looks at Chase.

Then, he looks at Blaze.

"YES! You are right!"
says Pop Pop.

"THAT'S MY CAT!"

CPSIA information can be obtained
at www.ICGtesting.com
Printed in the USA
BVHW062204310822
646040BV00004B/33